KU-587-382

South Dublin Libraries
www.southdublinlibraries.ie

TABLE OF CONTENTS

INTRODUCTION

Since what you devour could have a prime effect in your frame, digestive issues are fantastically not unusual.

Food is a not unusual trigger of digestive signs. Interestingly, restricting certain foods can dramatically enhance those signs in sensitive humans. In particular, an eating regimen low in fermentable carbs called FODMAPS is clinically endorsed for the control of irritable bowel syndrome (IBS).

FODMAPs are types of carbohydrates discovered in sure meals, which include wheat and beans. Studies have proven strong links between

FODMAPs and digestive signs like gasoline, bloating, stomach ache, diarrhea and constipation. Low-FODMAP diets can provide great benefits for plenty people with not unusual digestive disorders.

This cookbook gives tasty and easy recipes for FODMAPs and low-FODMAP diets with meal plans, how it works and who need to strive it.

WHAT ARE FODMAPS?

FODMAP stands for "fermentable oligo-, di-, mono-saccharides and polyols".

These are brief-chain carbs that are immune to digestion. Instead of being absorbed into your bloodstream, they attain the long way end of your gut in which maximum of your intestine bacteria reside.

Your intestine microorganism then use these carbs for fuel, producing hydrogen fuel and causing digestive signs and symptoms in touchy individuals. FODMAPs also draw liquid into your gut, which might also reason diarrhea.

Although now not anybody is touchy to FODMAPs, that is very not unusual amongst human beings with irritable bowel syndrome (IBS).

Common FODMAPs consist of:

- Fructose: An easy sugar found in lots of fruits and greens that still makes up the shape of desk sugar and most introduced sugars.

- Lactose: A carbohydrate discovered in dairy merchandise like milk.

- Fructans: Found in lots of foods, inclusive of grains like wheat, spelt, rye and barley.

South Dublin Libraries
www.southdublinlibraries.ie

- Galactans: Found in big amounts in legumes.

- Polyols: Sugar alcohols like xylitol, sorbitol, maltitol and mannitol. They are found in some end result and greens and frequently used as sweeteners.

FODMAP stands for "fermentable oligo-, di-, mono-saccharides and polyols." These are small carbs that many human beings cannot digest — specially people with irritable bowel syndrome (IBS).

WHAT EXPERT SAYS WITH RESEARCH CONDUCTED

The Low-FODMAP weight-reduction plan reduces certain carbohydrates to help relieve symptoms of IBS. There is great studies in this weight loss program's effectiveness. Because it involves keeping off sure meals, specialists agree it's helpful to work with an expert to maximize picks for lengthy-term use.

Several research help low FODMAP diets for coping with IBS signs. One 2014 scientific trial in comparison the effects of low FODMAP diets in human beings with and without IBS. The examine authors found that IBS signs stepped forward in the low FODMAP institution within a week of enforcing the food regimen.

People saw enhancements with abdominal ache, bloating, stool consistency, and flatulence. One 2016 document in Clinical and Experimental Gastroenterology, discovered that as much as 86% of humans with IBS noticed enhancements in their symptoms even as on a low FODMAP food regimen.

One present day 2017 file found that low FODMAP ingredients provide benefits for human beings with IBS. It additionally determined that sure traces and doses of probiotics may be beneficial, although extra research is wanted to identify the best options.

Another 2017 assessment concluded that low FODMAP diets offer favorable consequences for IBS signs and symptoms but did no longer discover that FODMAP diets are advanced to traditional diet plans for IBS.

HOW THE LOW FODMAP DIET WORKS

The low-FODMAP weight-reduction plan consists of very unique meals to keep away from and meals to eat. With every food organization, some foods are taken into consideration excessive in FODMAPs whilst others are low. For instance, apples and bananas are each fruits, however handiest the latter is taken into consideration low-FODMAP.

Some compliant foods on the low-FODMAP food plan encompass:

1. Fruit: Banana, blueberries, cantaloupe, str awberries, oranges, lemons, tomatoes, gr apes, and many others.

2. Vegetables: Carrots, bell   peppers, green beans, potatoes, squash, spinach, kale, eg gplant, and so on

3. Grains: Brown   rice,   oats,   quinoa, amaranth, bulgar, spelt, etc.

4. Nuts   and   seeds: chia   seeds, pumpkin seeds,   sesame   seeds, sunflower seeds, brazil

nuts, peanuts, pecans, walnuts, pine nuts, and macadamia nuts.

5. Animal

    products: beef, fowl, pork, eggs, turkey, fi sh, butter, lactose-loose milk, mozzarella cheese, etc.

6. Other: tofu, tempeh, almond milk, brown sugar, maple syrup, sugar, oils, herbs, spices, coffee, tea, and so forth.

Eating a low FODMAP food plan is a bit greater complicated than clearly warding off sure meals. This is because some foods contain better degrees of FODMAPs when they may be fed on in larger portions. Therefore, the form of food and quantity of meals are critical.

For example, fans can simplest eat ⅛ of an avocado at a time, and positive nuts need to be restricted to 10. Similarly, coconut milk have to be limited to ½ cup and bulgar ought to be restrained to ¼ cup cooked. Artificial sweeteners are allowed at the weight-reduction plan, but sugar alcohols aren't. Sugar alcohols generally result in -ol.

The listing of low-FODMAP ingredients is enormous, however so is that of high-FODMAP ingredients that must be averted. Some examples encompass watermelon, honey, excessive fructose corn syrup, most dairy merchandise, cauliflower, garlic, onions, asparagus, legumes, barley, rye, soy milk, pasta, etc.

WHO SHOULD FOLLOW A LOW-FODMAP DIET

A low-FODMAP diet isn't always for all and sundry. Unless you've got been recognized with IBS, studies suggests the food plan ought to do greater damage than suitable.

This is because maximum FODMAPs are prebiotics, which means they guide the increase of properly intestine microorganism.

Also, most of the research has been in adults. Therefore, there may be constrained help for the weight loss program in kids with IBS.

If you have IBS, take into account this weight loss program if you:

- Have ongoing intestine symptoms.

- Haven't spoken back to pressure management strategies.

- Haven't spoken back to first-line dietary recommendation, inclusive of proscribing alcohol, caffeine, highly spiced food and other common cause ingredients.

That said, there is a few hypothesis that the weight loss plan may advantage different situations, along with diverticulitis and exercising-precipitated digestive troubles. More research is underway.

It is essential to be conscious that the diet is a worried procedure. For this cause, it's no longer endorsed to try it for the primary time while visiting or during a busy or traumatic duration.

A low-FODMAP eating regimen is usually recommended for adults with IBS. The evidence for its use in other conditions is limited and may do more damage than properly.

HOW TO FOLLOW A LOW-FODMAP DIET

A low-FODMAP weight loss program is greater complicated than you might imagine and entails 3 degrees.

Stage 1: Restriction

This stage includes strict avoidance of all excessive-FODMAP foods. If you're not sure which foods are high in FODMAPs, read this book.

People who comply with this diet often suppose they should avoid all FODMAPs long-term, however this level must only final approximately three–eight weeks. This is as it's crucial to encompass FODMAPs inside the eating regimen for gut fitness.

Some human beings word an improvement in symptoms inside the first week, while others take the entire eight weeks. Once you've got ok relief of your digestive signs, you could development to the second level.

If with the aid of 8 weeks your intestine signs have now not resolved, confer with the What If Your Symptoms Don't Improve? Bankruptcy under.

Stage 2: Reintroduction

This degree includes systematically reintroducing excessive-FODMAP meals.

The reason of this is twofold:

1. To perceive which kinds of FODMAPs you tolerate. Few human beings are touchy to them all.

2. To set up the amount of FODMAPs you could tolerate. This is referred to as your "threshold degree."

In this step, you take a look at particular foods one after the other for three days every. It is suggested that you undertake this step with a trained dietitian who can guide you thru the suitable ingredients.

It is worth noting that you need to keep a low-FODMAP weight-reduction plan for the duration of this degree. This way even if you could tolerate a sure excessive-FODMAP food, you need to keep to restriction it until stage three. It is also essential to remember that, not like human beings with most meals hypersensitive reactions, human beings with IBS can tolerate small quantities of FODMAPs.

Lastly, despite the fact that digestive signs and symptoms may be debilitating, they will now not cause long-time period damage on your frame.

Stage 3: Personalization

This stage is also called the "changed low-FODMAP food plan." In different words, you still restriction a few FODMAPs. However, the quantity and type are tailor-made in your private tolerance, diagnosed in stage 2.

It is vital to development to this very last degree with a view to boom eating regimen range and versatility. These traits are connected with advanced lengthy-term compliance, first-class of lifestyles and intestine fitness.

Many people are surprised to discover that the low-FODMAP weight-reduction plan is a three-stage technique. Each stage is similarly vital in achieving long-time period symptom alleviation and standard health and nicely-being.

THREE THINGS TO DO BEFORE YOU GET STARTED

There are three stuff you have to do before embarking at the weight loss plan.

1. Make Sure You Actually Have IBS

Digestive signs can arise in lots of conditions, a few harmless and others extra serious.

Unfortunately, there's no positive diagnostic check to verify you've got IBS. For this cause, it's far endorsed you notice a doctor to rule out extra extreme conditions first, such as celiac disorder, inflammatory bowel sickness and colon most cancers.

Once those are dominated out, your medical doctor can affirm you have IBS using the legit IBS diagnostic criteria — you need to fulfill all three to be diagnosed with IBS:

Recurrent stomach ache: On common, at least at some point in keeping with week in the ultimate three months.

Stool signs: These should suit two or extra of the subsequent: associated with defecation, associated with a change in frequency of stool or related to a trade in the arrival of stool.

Persistent signs and symptoms: Criteria fulfilled for the remaining three months with symptom onset at least six months earlier than prognosis.

2. Try First-Line Diet Strategies

The low-FODMAP eating regimen is a time- and aid-intensive manner. This is why in medical practice it is taken into consideration 2nd-line dietary advice and is most effective used in a subset of human beings with IBS who don't respond to first-line strategies.

3. Plan Ahead

The food plan may be tough to comply with in case you aren't organized. Here are a few hints:

Find out what to shop for: Ensure you have get entry to credible low-FODMAP food lists. See under for a listing of where to locate these.

Get rid of high-FODMAP foods: Clear your refrigerator and pantry of these ingredients. Make a purchasing listing: Create a low-FODMAP shopping list before heading to the grocery store, so that you know which meals to purchase or keep away from.

Read menus in advance: Familiarize yourself with low-FODMAP menu alternatives so that you'll be prepared while eating out.

Before you embark at the low-FODMAP diet, there are several belongings you want to do. These easy steps will help growth your probabilities of efficiently coping with your digestive symptoms.

BENEFITS OF A LOW-FODMAP DIET

A low-FODMAP weight loss plan restricts excessive-FODMAP ingredients. The benefits of a low-FODMAP diet were tested in lots of humans with IBS throughout greater than 30 research.

Reduced Digestive Symptoms

IBS digestive signs and symptoms can vary widely, along with belly pain, bloating, reflux, flatulence and bowel urgency.

Stomach pain is a hallmark of the situation, and bloating has been discovered to have an effect on extra than 80% of human beings with IBS.

Needless to mention, these signs can be debilitating. One big look at even stated that human beings with IBS stated they might give up a median of 25% in their final lives to be symptom-unfastened.

Fortunately, each belly pain and bloating have been shown to seriously lower with a low-FODMAP food plan.

Evidence from four amazing research concluded that in case you follow a low-FODMAP food plan, your odds of enhancing belly pain and bloating are eighty one% and 75% more, respectively. Several different studies have recommended the eating regimen can help manage flatulence, diarrhea and constipation.

Increased Quality of Life

People with IBS regularly record a reduced best of life, and intense digestive signs had been associated with this.

Luckily, several studies have located the low-FODMAP diet improves typical excellent of existence. There is also a few evidence showing that a low-FODMAP food plan may additionally boom electricity stages in humans with IBS, but placebo-managed research are needed to aid this finding.

There is convincing proof for the blessings of a low-FODMAP weight-reduction plan. The food regimen appears to improve digestive symptoms in approximately 70% of adults with IBS.

FOODS TO EAT

Low-FODMAP Vegetables

There are some dozen compliant vegetables on the low-FODMAP weight loss program. Some of them encompass potatoes, sweet potatoes, eggplant, collard veggies, cabbage, kale, lettuce, squash, bell peppers, carrots, bok choy, arugula, and turnips.

Low-FODMAP Fruit

What makes a fruit low-FODMAP is that it's low in fructose and fructans, which may cause bloating and gas in excessive quantities. Some low-FODMAP fruits encompass bananas, blueberries, grapes, kiwis, lemons, raspberries, strawberries, oranges, pineapple, cantaloupe, and honeydew melon.

Low-FODMAP Grains

Many people anticipate that grains are off-limits on the low-FODMAP eating regimen. While a few are, you can still experience amaranth, brown rice, oats, quinoa, spelt, and small quantities of bulgar. Some of those grains contain gluten.

Because many grains that contain gluten, also happen to be high FODMAP foods, which include wheat, rye, and barley, many human beings discover comfort of signs and symptoms while following a gluten-unfastened weight loss plan, despite the fact that a strict gluten-loose eating regimen might not necessary for all, until a person also has celiac sickness or non-celiac gluten sensitivity

Most Nuts and Seeds

Nuts and seeds are super snacks and exceptional resources of vitamins and wholesome fats. Most nuts and seeds are within the clean. Some consist of chia seeds, pumpkin seeds, sesame seeds, sunflower seeds, Brazil nuts, peanuts, pecans, walnuts, pine nuts, and macadamia nuts.

Certain Sweeteners

Many sweeteners are high in fructans and fructose, which ought to be constrained whilst following the low-FODMAP weight loss program. Compliant sweeteners encompass white sugar, brown sugar, maple syrup, powdered sugar, and a few synthetic sweeteners. Sweeteners ought to be used sparingly in any food regimen.

Most Non-Dairy Milk

Since the low-FODMAP weight loss plan is nearly dairy-free, you could update your milk products with non-dairy alternatives. The ones which can be low-FODMAP are almond milk, hemp milk, rice milk, and small quantities of coconut milk.

Lactose-Free Dairy Products

Lactose is the main cause why most dairy products are considered excessive-FODMAP.

Lactose-loose dairy merchandise are compliant, though. Look for milk, ice lotions, and yogurts which are freed from lactose. Some cheeses, inclusive of mozzarella and Parmesan, are also allowed on a low-FODMAP food plan.

Meat, Fish, and Eggs

All different animal merchandise except dairy are allowed on the low-FODMAP food regimen. This consists of red meat, chicken, pork, eggs, turkey, and seafood. However, some researchers advocate keeping off processed meats like sausage.

Tofu and Tempeh

Followers of the low-FODMAP food regimen can use tofu and tempeh as resources of protein. The low-FODMAP eating regimen isn't always soy-unfastened, although soy milk is not encouraged. Vegans and vegetarians are especially encouraged to devour tofu and tempeh in location of legumes to satisfy their protein requirements.

FOODS TO AVOID

High-FODMAP Vegetables

Some veggies are believed to purpose fuel, bloating, and different digestive signs and symptoms because of their excessive-FODMAP content. Some examples encompass artichokes, garlic, onions, leeks, asparagus, beets, cauliflower, mushrooms, Brussels sprouts, celery, and peas.

High-FODMAP Fruit

Fruits are acknowledged for their herbal sugar content material. Some of the sweetest fruits can motive uncomfortable digestive troubles due to those sugars. On the low-FODMAP diet, lessen your intake of apples, cherries, mangoes, peaches, pears, watermelon, and apricots. You ought to additionally avoid canned fruit, dried fruit, and fruit juice that's high in fructose.

High-FODMAP Grains

There are a handful of high-FODMAP grains that have to be prevented. Barley, couscous, faro, rye, wheat, and semolina are a number of them. Make certain that any cereals, pasta, bread, and crackers you devour are free of these grains.

Legumes

Beans are a commonplace wrongdoer of many unwanted digestive signs, such as fuel. There's a systematic explanation, too. Legumes are excessive in galactooligosaccharides (GOS), which belong to the FODMAP circle of relatives. They can reason bloating, stomach pain, and different IBS symptoms. Avoid all legumes, which include beans, lentils, and pulses.

Some Nuts

Most nuts are low-FODMAP, however there are some which can be high in FODMAPs and have to be restricted. This consists of almonds, cashews, hazelnuts, and pistachios. However, a few specialists recommend that almonds and hazelnuts may be fed on in very small amounts (10 or fewer nuts) in some humans.

Certain Sweeteners

As you may consider, some sweeteners are excessive in fructans and fructose, which can be a part of the FODMAP circle of relatives. Some of the ones you ought to keep away from consist of honey, agave nectar, high fructose corn syrup, molasses, isomalt, and sugar alcohols, such as erythritol, isomalt, lactitol, maltitol, mannitol, sorbitol, and xylitol.

Most Dairy Products

The low-FODMAP weight loss program is nearly dairy-free. Lactose is a commonplace trigger for human beings with IBS and IBD, so lactose-containing ingredients should be avoided. This consists of cow's milk, goat's milk, soft cheeses, yogurt, ice cream, and buttermilk.

Some Non-dairy Milk

Oat milk and soy milk are among a number of the few non-dairy kinds of milk which might be considered high-FODMAP. Switch to a low-FODMAP milk alternative that's high in vitamins. Be careful of non-dairy sorts of milk with added FODMAPs, together with artificial sweeteners and excessive-fructose corn syrup.

IS A LOW-FODMAP DIET NUTRITIONALLY BALANCED?

You can nonetheless meet your nutritional requirements on a low-FODMAP weight loss program. However, like several restrictive weight loss plan, you have an extended danger of dietary deficiencies.

In particular, you need to be aware of your fiber and calcium intake at the same time as on a low-FODMAP weight loss program.

Fiber

Many ingredients which can be high in fiber also are excessive in FODMAPs. Therefore, people frequently lessen their fiber intake on a low-FODMAP weight loss plan.

This may be averted through changing high-FODMAP, high-fiber meals like culmination and vegetables with low-FODMAP types that also offer lots of dietary fiber.

Low-FODMAP sources of fiber consist of oranges, raspberries, strawberries, green beans, spinach, carrots, oats, brown rice, quinoa, gluten-unfastened brown bread and flaxseeds.

Calcium

Dairy meals are an excellent supply of calcium. However, many dairy meals are limited on a low-FODMAP eating regimen. This is why your calcium consumption might also lower while following this weight loss program.

Low-FODMAP assets of calcium encompass hard and elderly cheese, lactose-free milk and yogurt, canned fish with edible bones and calcium-fortified nuts, oats and rice milks.

A low-FODMAP weight-reduction plan may be nutritionally balanced. However, there may be a chance of a few dietary deficiencies, which includes fiber and calcium.

RECOMMENDED TIMING

There isn't a reliable endorsed number of food in line with at the low-FODMAP eating regimen. However, the usual is three food in keeping with day—breakfast, lunch, and dinner—with mild snacking in-among.

I recommend spacing out food by way of 3 to four hours. If possible, go away multiple hours in-between snacks and food.

Some other pointers include:

1. Consume constrained fruit, especially in the identical meal.

2. Get a variety of meals in place of ingesting the identical food again and again. Since the weight loss program is already restrictive, make sure to eat a variety of compliant foods to maximize nutrient consumption.

3. Make water your most important beverage. Though coffee and a few teas are allowed, water can assist move stools less difficult via the digestive tract.

4. Limit alcohol consumption.

CAN VEGETARIANS FOLLOW A LOW-FODMAP DIET?

A nicely-balanced vegetarian eating regimen may be low in FODMAPs. Nonetheless, following a low-FODMAP food plan if you are a vegetarian can be more difficult.

This is because high-FODMAP legumes are staple protein ingredients in vegetarian diets. That said, you may include small quantities of canned and rinsed legumes in a low-FODMAP eating regimen. Serving sizes are usually approximately 1/4 cup (64 grams).

There also are many low-FODMAP, protein-wealthy options for vegetarians, along with tempeh, tofu, eggs, Quorn (a meat substitute) and most nuts and seeds.

There are many protein-rich vegetarian options appropriate for an extremely low-FODMAP diet. Therefore, there may be no reason why a vegetarian with IBS can't follow a nicely-balanced low-FODMAP weight loss plan.

LOW FODMAP RECIPES

Low FODMAP Buffalo Chicken Dip

Ingredients

Serves 6

- 12 oz. Boneless hen breasts, cooked and shredded

- ¼ cup warm sauce (without garlic, onion such as Texas Petes)

- 1 cup Green Valley lactose unfastened sour cream

- 1 cup Green valley lactose unfastened cream cheese

- 2 cups shredded Cheddar cheese

- ¼ chopped cup green onion/scallions (green element only)

Instructions

1. Preheat oven to 350 degrees F.

2. Combine shredded hen, warm sauce, bitter cream, cream cheese, 1 1/2 cups of the Cheddar cheese and a pair of tablespoons of the green onion.

3. Spread dip right into a small casserole dish and top with remaining cheddar cheese.

4. Bake for 25 mins or until dip is excellent and bubbly.

5. Garnish with last inexperienced onion.

6. Serve with child carrots, bell peppers strips, and corn tortilla chips!

Low FODMAP Antipasto Skewers

Ingredients

Recipe may be adjusted to your wishes

Serving length 2-3 skewers

- 1 small jar peperoncini

- 1 small jar pitted Kalamata olives

- 1 small container clean small mozzarella balls

- Thinly sliced prosciutto, reduce in thirds lengthwise

- Fresh basil leaves, washed and sliced in half

- 1 small field grape tomatoes

- small bamboo skewers approximately 6 inches lengthy

Instructions

1. If pepperoncini are large, reduce in half

2. Fold prosciutto into layered square to healthy on skewer.

3. Thread ingredients on skewer as preferred.

4. Serve on platter!

Lemon Parsley Roasted Shrimp

Ingredients

- 1 pound greater big shrimp (peeled and de-veined, can leave tail shell on, if desired)

- 2 tablespoons garlic infused oil

- 2 tablespoons lemon juice

- 1/2 teaspoon overwhelmed pink pepper flakes

- sea salt and pepper, to taste

- 1/4 cup shredded Parmesan

- 1/4 freshly chopped parsley

Instructions

1. Preheat oven to 400 tiers F.

2. Lightly oil cookie sheet.

3. Pat shrimp dry with paper towel and add
   to cookie sheet in even layer.

4. In small bowl, whisk together oil, lemon,
   beaten red pepper, sea salt and pepper,
   to taste and drizzle evenly over shrimp.

5. Roast shrimp for 6-eight mins, until
   cooked thru and opaque.

6. Remove shrimp from oven and sprinkle
   with shredded Parmesan and sparkling
   parsley.

Parmesan Roasted Broccoli

Ingredients

Serves 4

- 3 cups broccoli florets

- 2 eggs

- 1/3 cup Parmesan cheese

- 1/3 cup almond flour (I used Bob's Red Mill first-rate-first-class almond flour)

Instructions

1. Preheat oven to 350 tiers F and lightly oil baking sheet.

2. In small bowl, whisk both eggs to combination.

3. On large plate or in a plastic bag, mix Parmesan and almond flour.

4. Dip approximately 1 broccoli florets in egg, then upload to Parmesan and almond flour aggregate to lightly coat.

5. Place broccoli on baking sheet. Repeat technique with last broccoli.

6. Place in oven and bake for 15-20 mins. Turn broccoli during mid-point of cooking time.

Orange Cranberry Walnut Scones (gluten loose + low FODMAP)

Ingredients

Serving length: 2 mini scones or one medium sized scone.

Yield: 16 mini scones; 12 medium scones.

- 2 cups gluten loose flour mixture (along with King Arthur GF measure for measure or Bob's Red Mill GF 1 for 1)

- 1 1/2 teaspoon baking powder (use gluten unfastened if following gluten loose food regimen)

- half of teaspoon baking soda

- half cup sugar

- 1 massive egg

- 1/4 cup sour cream (this can provide minimal lactose per serving)

- 12 tablespoons bloodless unsalted butter

- 2 teaspoons orange zest

- 1/4 cup dried cranberries, finely chopped

- 1/4 cup walnuts, finely chopped

Orange glaze:

- 2/3 cup confectioner's sugar

- 1 teaspoon orange zest

- 1 1/2 tablespoons freshly squeezed orange juice

Instructions

1. Preheat oven to four hundred stages F.

2. Prepare scone pan if the use of or add parchment paper to baking sheet.

3. In big bowl, add flour combo, baking powder, soda and sugar. Set aside.

4. In small bowl, mix egg and sour cream, set aside.

5. Slice butter in chew length pieces and add to flour aggregate. Using pastry blender or palms, mix butter into flour mixture until the mixture resembles direction crumbs.

6. Add sour cream and egg combination to flour mixture.

7. Fold in orange zest, cranberries and walnuts.

8. If the use of mini scone pan, add dough frivolously to pan. If making scones into rounds, divide dough in half. Make 2 small rounds along with your arms. Cut every spherical into 6 triangular fashioned scones (like slicing a pie) and place scones on baking sheet approximately an inch apart.

9. Bake scones for 15 minutes. The scones need to be gently browned on the edges.

10. While scones cool, make orange glaze. Simply add confectioner's sugar, zest and

orange juice and blend with a fork until combined. Drizzle over scones.

Chocolate Avocado Waffles

Ingredients

- Makes 4 waffles--serving length 1 waffle

- 2 tablespoons ripe avocado, mashed

- 1/4 cup cocoa (I used Hershey's Cocoa--special dark)

- 1 big egg

- 1 cup Gluten Free Waffle Mix (I used my DIY Low FODMAP & Gluten Free Waffle Mix-seek my blog)

- 2/3 cup lactose free milk

- 2 tablespoons semi-candy chocolate morsels

- Dress up with butter, strawberry slices and sprinkle of confectioner's sugar

Instructions

1. Prepare waffle maker by using lightly oiling and heating as directed.

2. In medium bowl, upload mashed avocado, cocoa powder and egg, mixing to combo.

3. Add in waffle mix and milk, stirring till mixture is clean.

4. Fold in semi-sweet chocolate morsels.

5. Pour batter into waffle maker and cook as directed on waffle maker (times may also range depending on length of waffles)

6. Dress up waffles with butter, strawberry slices and confectioner's sugar, as preferred.

DIY Low FODMAP & Gluten Free Waffle Mix

Ingredients

Makes approximately 3 half of cup of waffle blend (can double recipe)

- 3 cups gluten loose flour

- 1/3 cup sugar

- 1 half teaspoons baking powder (use gluten loose if following gluten free food plan)

- 1 teaspoon baking soda

- half teaspoon salt

Instructions

1. Add the gluten free flour combination, sugar, baking powder, baking soda and salt into a large glass Mason jar or comparable sealed container.

To make 4 waffles:

2. In medium bowl, add 1 cup of waffle blend, 1 egg, 1 half of tablespoons

vegetable oil or melted butter, 2/3 cup of

lactose unfastened milk

Gluten Free Egg and Cheese Soufflé

Ingredients

This recipe is gluten free but does comprise trace

ability FODMAPs in Worcestershire sauce

- five Slices Udi's GF bread (White sandwich

  bread is low FODMAP)

- 2 tablespoons butter

- 4 eggs

- 2 cups milk (use lactose free if lactose

  intolerance)

- 1 cup preferred GF cheese (cheddar, pepper jack works well)

- 1 ½ tsp. Lea and Perrin's Worcestershire Sauce (It's GF too)

- 1 ½ tsp. Yellow mustard (check elements to ensure its GF mustard)

- 1-2 tsp. Sparkling chives, finely chopped

Instructions

Butter bread and reduce into cubes (about 6 cubes in step with slice.)

3. Add buttered bread cubes to 8 x 8 casserole dish or 9 inch round casserole

4. Whip eggs, milk, Worcestershire sauce and mustard together.

5. Pour egg combination over bread, cover tightly with plastic wrap and refrigerate overnight.

6. Preheat oven to 350 levels and bake for 55 mins till cooked thru and barely browned on pinnacle.

Hash Brown Egg Nests

Ingredients

- 4 cups shredded hash brown potatoes (uncooked) I used plain frozen shredded-fashion hash browns that I defrosted. You could also strive grating 2-3 huge peeled uncooked Yukon Gold or similar potatoes for an alternative.

- 2 egg whites

- 1 tablespoon garlic infused oil or simple olive oil

- salt and pepper

- 12 eggs (big)

- 1 medium zucchini or summer season squash, trimmed and very thinly sliced (for quick cooking)

- 1 cup shredded cheddar cheese

- 6 slices of cooked bacon, if preferred. Cut each slice into chew size portions.

- Garnish w/ clean chopped parsley and pepper, if favored.

Instructions

1. Preheat oven to 425 levels F.

2. Generously oil, muffin tin for 12.

3. In medium bowl, upload potatoes, egg whites, garlic infused oil, sprint of salt and pepper. (If using clean grated potatoes, be sure to strain off any liquid.)

4. Gently fold egg whites and oil into potatoes.

5. Divide potato mixture frivolously into the 12 muffin cups.

6. Press potato mixture firmly into each muffin cup, allowing some potatoes to line the internal of the muffin (forming a crust)

7. Place muffin tin in oven for 15 minutes to bake potatoes. Remove.

8. Top each of the potato crusts with a few slices of squash and a sprinkle of cheese, calmly.

9. Crack an egg, and upload it on top of the squash and cheese.

10. Add bacon to the pinnacle of the egg, if favored.

11. Return muffin tin to the oven and bake for 15-20 mins or till egg is ready and cooked via.

12. Garnish w/ parsley and pepper, if preferred.

Kale, publisher 1st baron verulam, Tomato Egg White Omelet in a Mug

Ingredients

- 4 egg whites, lightly beaten (If using boxed egg whites that is three/4 cup) OR use 2 whole eggs alternatively.

- 2 tablespoons completely cooked ham or hen bacon, in chew length pieces (I use the al fresco fowl bacon, 1 strip consistent with mug)

- 2 tablespoons clean infant kale or spinach, sliced (I used kale)

- 2 tablespoon tomato, diced

- 1 tablespoon shredded cheddar cheese

- Dash of oregano or basil, if preferred

- salt and pepper to taste, if favored

Instructions

1. Lightly oil the inner of espresso mug.

2. Toss the elements inside the mug and stir (ingredients need to fill mug about 3/4 complete)

3. Pop into the microwave and prepare dinner for 1 minute. Check for doneness-- will possibly need every other minute of cooking time to ensure the egg is cooked and cheese is melted.

4. Enjoy.

Low FODMAP German Pancake with Berries

Ingredients

- 1/4 cup oat flour

- 1/4 cup gluten unfastened flour combination (I used King Arthur GF multipurpose flour)

- 3 big eggs, whisked

- half cup lactose unfastened milk

- 1 tablespoon sugar

- 1/4 teaspoon vanilla or almond extract, optional

Garnish:

- A few sliced strawberries, handful of blueberries, butter, sprinkle of confectioner's sugar, as favored.

Instructions

1. Preheat oven to 450 ranges F.

2. Lightly grease your cast iron skillet (9 or 11 inch will paintings)

3. In medium bowl, mix the flours, eggs, milk, sugar and extract with a fork, till just blended and freed from any lumps.

4. Pour aggregate into solid iron skillet. Bake for 12 minutes or till edges are lightly brown and pancake is overvalued.

5. Remove from oven, garnish with toppings as desired.

6. Eat at once.

One Pan Breakfast: Hash Browns, Eggs, Avocado & Tomato

Ingredients

Serves 6

- 2 teaspoons oil (grapeseed, canola, safflower)

- 6 cups shredded potato (I used frozen without any onion or garlic)

- 6 pre-cooked sausage hyperlinks or patties or pre-cooked bacon strips-- without FODMAP components-- tear or cut bacon into chunk size pieces.

- 6 huge eggs

- 8 cherry tomatoes, halved

- half yellow bell pepper, deseeded and sliced

- half teaspoon taco seasoning (I used FODY brand)

- 1/4 cup shredded cheddar cheese, non-obligatory

- half of avocado, sliced into chunk size portions

- 2 tablespoons, sparkling chopped cilantro or parsley, non-compulsory

- 1-2 inexperienced scallions/spring onion(s), inexperienced part best, sliced

Instructions

1. Preheat oven to 375 stages F.

2. On rimmed baking sheet, drizzle oil over backside.

3. Add potatoes and if using frozen sausage links, add in now. Bake for 20-25 minutes, stirring a few times for the duration of cooking time, until hash browns are gently browned (and sausages are warmed thru).

4. Remove baking sheet from oven.

5. Crack each egg personally into small dish and region cautiously over potatoes.

6. Scatter tomatoes and bell pepper over potatoes.

7. If the usage of pre-cooked bacon, add in now.

8. Season top of eggs with taco seasoning.

9. Place baking sheet returned into oven for 5-10 minute or until eggs are set.

10. Remove from oven and garnish dish with cilantro or parsley (if desired), avocado and green onion.

Sweet Potato & a Sunny Side

Ingredients

Serves 2

1. 1 cup thinly sliced washed sweet potato, skin intact (approximately 1/2 medium)

2. 1 teaspoon olive oil

3. 2 large entire eggs

4. 1/4 cup infant spinach &/or kale, sliced

5. salt and pepper, to taste

Instructions

1. Using mandoline slicer, cut candy potato thinly.

2. In medium skillet, add oil and heat over medium heat.

3. Layer potatoes frivolously in 2 circles, overlapping potatoes.

4. Cook potatoes for about 5 mins or till lightly browned, then turn them over.

5. Add one egg to each sweet potato 'circle', and lightly cowl skillet cooking egg, approximately three-five minutes.

6. Remove cover, add spinach &/or kale, and season with salt and pepper.

7. Using spatula, carefully switch to plate.

Lemon Arugula Pesto with Macadamias

Ingredients

- 4 cups basil leaves, washed and trimmed

- 1 cup infant arugula

- 1/3-1/2 cup sparkling lemon juice (I used the half cup because I LOVE lemon!)

- 1/2 cup salted macadamias

- 1/2 cup Parmesan cheese

- 1 garlic or (FODMAPers--use 1 TB of your garlic infused oil)

- Salt/pepper to flavor

Instructions

1. In a food processor match with metallic blade, add all the elements and mix for about 2 mins.

2. Mixture ought to have some texture but usual be at the smooth size.

3. Options for use: I introduced 2 TB of the pesto to a few cups of infant arugula. I brought a bit creamy goat cheese on the

lowest of my plate, crowned with a serving of the dressed arugula and crowned with a few sautéed prosciutto and a few sliced tomatoes. Alternatively you may brush some of the pesto on grilled chook (grill fowl first and brush pesto on whilst nonetheless warm) or use instead of tomato sauce on a pizza crust.

Homemade BBQ Sauce (FODMAP-friendly)

Ingredients

South Dublin Libraries
www.southdublinlibraries.ie

- 1 14.5 ounce can diced tomatoes

- 1 Tablespoon Maille Dijon Mustard

- 1 Tablespoon Rice wine vinegar

- 2 Tablespoons Brown Sugar

- half of teaspoon paprika

- dash of McCormick's Gourmet Collection Chipotle Chili Pepper (non-obligatory)

- 1 teaspoon Garlic-infused oil

- 1/2 cup grated carrots

- salt and pepper to flavor

Instructions

1. In medium saucepan over medium warmth upload all the ingredients besides salt and pepper.

2. Simmer sauce for approximately five minutes, stirring every so often.

3. Shut off warmth and allow calm down for a few minutes. Taste and season for your liking.

4. Carefully add on your blender whilst now not warm but slightly heat.

5. Blend for a couple of minutes to easy consistency.

6. For pulled chook, simmer sauce with 2 boneless skinless chicken breasts and half cup of water over medium low warmth for half-hour or till hen is cooked via. (Add greater water as important--sauce must continue to be sauce-like now not dried out!

7. Shred hen using 2 forks to drag chicken apart.

Berry Cobbler (gluten unfastened + low FODMAP)

Ingredients

Serves 6

Berry aggregate:

- 1 cup blueberries (sparkling or frozen)

- 2 1/2 cup small to medium length strawberries (clean or frozen)

- 2 teaspoons sugar

- Juice of one lemon

- 1 tablespoon GF flour

- Cobbler topping

- 1 cup gluten loose flour blend

- half cup sugar

- 1 teaspoon vanilla

- 2/3 cup lactose free milk

- 3 tablespoons melted butter

- 1 teaspoon baking powder (pick out a GF logo if following GF diet)

- 1 egg

- 1-2 scoops appropriate low lactose ice cream

- 1/4 cup chopped walnuts

Instructions

1. Preheat oven to 350 tiers F.

2. In 10 inch forged iron skillet or pie plate, upload berries, 1 teaspoon sugar, lemon juice and 1 tablespoon GF flour, stir to mix.

3. In medium bowl, upload 1 cup GF flour mixture, half cup sugar, lactose unfastened milk, melted butter, baking powder and egg. Blend collectively with fork until consistency of pancake batter.

4. Add cobbler aggregate over top of berries by way of the spoonful, leaving some berries exposed.

5. Place in oven and bake for 20-half-hour. (Frozen berries will take in the direction of 30 minutes while sparkling berry mixture will prepare dinner among 20-25 mins).

6. Garnish with a couple scoops of appropriate ice cream and chopped walnuts if favored.

Coconut Milk Soft Serve "Ice Cream"

Ingredients

1. half of cup frozen unsweetened coconut milk

2. splash of coconut milk or water

3. 1 TB packed brown sugar

4. 1 tsp. Vanilla extract

5. Handful mini chocolate chips (chopped walnuts might be first-class too!)

Instructions

1. Freeze coconut milk in ice cube tray for several hours till frozen.

2. Add frozen coconut milk to blender and add in brown sugar and vanilla.

3. Add a touch of coconut milk to blender to 'skinny' out aggregate for the proper consistency.

4. Sprinkle some mini chocolate chips on pinnacle if preferred.

Baked low FODMAP Eggplant Parmesan

Ingredients

- 1 large eggplant, reduce in half of inch thick slices, ends trimmed (about 12 slices)

- salt

- 2 big eggs

- 1 cup plain gluten free breadcrumbs

- 1 tablespoon garlic infused oil (I used FODY meals emblem)

- 1 teaspoon dried basil

- 1 teaspoon dried oregano

- 1 half of cup diced undeniable canned tomatoes (tired of juice, without any onion or garlic ingredients)

- 2 tablespoons Parmesan cheese

- 1 cup grated mozzarella cheese

Instructions

1. Layer paper towels onto the lowest of a big rimmed baking sheet.

2. Layer eggplant slices on paper towel in unmarried layer and gently salt them to assist launch extra moisture. Let sit down for approximately 20-half-hour. Add a paper towel on top to acquire moisture from the tops.

3. Preheat oven to 375 levels F, while assembling the eggplant.

4. Transfer eggplant onto a plate.

5. Remove paper towels from baking sheet and dry baking sheet with towel.

6. Add a mild coating of oil to the baking sheet.

7. Next, whisk eggs in medium size bowl.

8. In every other medium length bowl or plate, add bread crumbs, 1/2 teaspoon basil and half of teaspoon oregano; stir to mix.

9. Add every eggplant slice (one at a time) into egg to coat on each facets, then add into breadcrumbs to coat each aspects. Press eggplant into breadcrumbs to help them stick.

10. Place every breaded eggplant slice onto baking sheet in a unmarried layer.

11. Place eggplant in the oven for 15 minutes to brown up and cook dinner, turning eggplant slices over at mid-cooking time.

12. While eggplant is cooking, add diced tomatoes, garlic infused oil, and half of teaspoon basil and 1/2 teaspoon oregano into small bowl; stir to blend.

13. Remove eggplant from oven, and flippantly distribute tomato sauce onto pinnacle of breaded eggplant.

14. Cover tomato sauce with grated Parmesan and mozzarella cheese.

15. Return to oven to melt cheese and heat up sauce-about 5 mins.

16. Enjoy!

Lobster Rangoons (lactose free, low FODMAP)

Ingredients

- Makes 30 stuffed wontons, serving size 6-8 lobster stuffed wontons

- 8 oz Green Valley Creamery lactose unfastened cream cheese

- 1 teaspoon lemon zest

- 1 teaspoon fresh squeezed lemon juice

- 1/4 cup chopped scallions (inexperienced element best)

- half pound cooked lobster meat, finely chopped

- 1 package deal of square wontons

- Fresh scallion veggies and lemon wedges as garish, if favored.

Instructions

1. Preheat oven to 375ºF. Mist baking sheet with cooking spray.

2. Mix together cream cheese, lemon zest and juice, and chopped scallions in a medium bowl. Stir in lobster meat.

3. Place a wonton wrapper on a flat floor. Cover remaining wrappers with a damp paper towel and set a bowl of water close by.

4. Place 1 heaping teaspoon of the lobster and cream cheese combination within the center of the wrapper.

5. Dip your finger in water and run along the edges of the wonton wrapper.

6. Fold the wrapper in half, making a triangle. Press down along the rims to seal and cast off any air trapped inside the wonton.

7. Place wonton on organized baking sheet, and repeat until you have 30 stuffed wontons.

8. Once assembled, mist lobster rangoons lightly with olive oil cooking spray.

9. Bake for 15 - 20 minutes (or until browned).

10. Serve straight away, garnish with chopped scallions and a lemon wedge, if preferred

Cheesy Turkey Tostada Pizzas (low FODMAP)

Ingredients

- 1 pound lean ground meat (hen breast, turkey, beef and so forth)

- 2 teaspoon ground chili powder (

- 1 teaspoon ground cumin, or extra to flavor

- 1 cup diced tomatoes or clean chopped, tired of juice

- Salt and pepper, to flavor

- 10 tostado shells

- 1 cup grated sharp or low-fat cheddar cheese

- 2 scallions, finely chopped (FODMAP followers use inexperienced component simplest)

Instructions

1. Preheat oven to 350 degrees

2. In big non-stick skillet over medium warmth, upload meat. (May want to feature a TB oil if meat is specially lean)

3. Cook meat, crumbling and stirring for approximately eight-10 mins.

4. Add chili powder, cumin, and tomatoes to the skillet. Reduce warmth and cook dinner for any other five mins or until

meat is thoroughly cooked. Season with a bit of salt and pepper if desired.

5. On a huge cookie sheet, unfold out tostada shells (some may overlap a small amount). Divide meat mixture evenly among tostadas.

6. Sprinkle cheddar frivolously over meat. Bake for 8-10 minutes.

7. Sprinkle with scallions, if preferred.

8. Serve with an aspect salad and a 1-2 slices of avocado

Pumpkin Spinach Stuffed Shells

Ingredients

Serves three-four; approximately 5-6 shells in keeping with character

- 18 large pasta gluten loose shells

- 1 1/2 cups lactose loose cottage cheese (I used lactaid brand)

- 1 cup canned pumpkin (not pumpkin pie filling)

- 2 tablespoons garlic infused oil

- 1 cup fresh spinach, packed, then chopped (you could sub in basil or use half of cup of basil and spinach as another option)

- 1/2 cup plus 2 tablespoons Parmesan cheese, grated

- 1 egg, overwhelmed

- salt and pepper, to flavor

- 1 half of cup finely chopped canned/boxed tomatoes (I used Pomi logo; choose brand without onion and garlic)

- 1/4 teaspoon basil

- 1/4 teaspoon oregano

- half cup shredded component skim mozzarella cheese

- Sliced fresh basil or spinach for garnish, elective

Instructions

1. Cook pasta in step with bundle directions.

2. While pasta is cooking, put together shell filling. In medium bowl, upload and mix lactose unfastened cottage cheese, canned pumpkin, 1 tablespoon garlic infused oil, and spinach or basil (or blend of each), half cup parmesan cheese, one egg & salt and pepper, to flavor. Set aside.

3. In medium bowl, add tomatoes, the other tablespoon of garlic infused oil, basil, oregano and blend; set aside.

4. When pasta is cooked (should be al dente), rinse well.

5. Preheat oven to 350 ranges.

6. In 8 x 8 pan, upload approximately 2/three of the tomato sauce combination to bottom of pan.

7. Start filling each pasta shell with about 1 - 1 half of tablespoon of cheese spinach combination; while shell is stuffed upload to rectangular pan with the filling facet up. Repeat with remaining shells.

8. Drizzle the rest of the tomato sauce over shells, pinnacle with the last Parmesan cheese, and mozzarella cheese.

9. Cover pan with aluminum foil and bake for 15-20 mins. Remove foil, go back to oven and cook dinner for another 5-10 mins until sauce is gently bubbling and the cheese is melted.

10. Sprinkle top with sliced basil or spinach, if favored.

11. Enjoy!

Prosciutto Carbonara with Kale (gluten loose + low FODMAP)

Ingredients

- 2 tablespoons greater virgin olive oil

- 3 ounces prosciutto, sliced in chew size strips

- 2 huge eggs, plus 2 egg yolks

- 1/4 cup Parmesan or Romano cheese, grated

- 12 ounces suitable gluten loose pasta (I used garafalo's casarecce)

- 1 cup sliced kale, stems eliminated or use infant kale

- Garnish and season with salt, pepper, crushed crimson pepper flakes, as desired.

Instructions

1. Boil beyond according to package deal guidelines-minus 1 minute of the suggested cooking time.

2. As pasta is cooking, add 1 tablespoon olive oil into huge skillet over medium warmness with prosciutto to lightly brown up, eliminate from warmness.

3. Remove proscuitto onto plate.

4. When pasta is performed, shop approximately 1 cup of the pasta water and stress pasta.

5. Add eggs and yolks to small bowl, add cheese, 1/4 cup warm pasta water and whisk together.

6. Add remaining oil to large skillet, put heat on low.

7. Add pasta and egg combination to skillet. Stir to combination. Add the remaining pasta water until you create a light 'sauce'.

8. Add kale to simply cook gently so it is gentle but still vivid green.

9. Add prosciutto and fold in to mixture.

10. Garnish as favored!

One Skillet Mexican Chicken & Rice Fiesta!

Ingredients

6 servings

- 1 pound ground chicken breast (can sub in floor beef or ground turkey)

- 1/4 cup suitable low FODMAP Taco Seasoning or blend 2 1/2 tablespoons chili powder (without onion or garlic), 1 half tablespoons cumin and 1/four teaspoon salt; upload a dash of cayenne pepper for a few warmness if you tolerate it

- 1, 14 ounce can diced tomatoes (fire roasted or undeniable; no onion or garlic), undrained

- 1 cup frozen plain corn niblets (optional)

- 3/4 cup lengthy grain rice

- 2 cups low FODMAP hen broth or water (I use homemade hen broth)

- 1 half cup shredded Colby jack cheese

Toppings:

- Lactose loose sour cream or small amount simple Greek yogurt, to your tolerance

- Diced avocado (limit to one/8 avocado consistent with serving)

- Sliced black olives

- Chopped clean cilantro

- Chopped scallions (inexperienced component handiest)

Instructions

1. In huge skillet over medium warmth, brown up floor hen, till not crimson.

2. Add in taco seasoning, diced tomatoes with juice, corn (if using), rice and hen broth or water.

3. Raise heat to excessive to carry aggregate to a boil, then lessen to simmer for 20 minutes, area cowl over skillet. Stir 1/2 manner thru cooking time.

4. Add cheese frivolously over top of meat mixture, replace cover for two-three mins or till cheese melts.

5. Add various toppings as favored.

One Skillet Shrimp, Tomato & Feta Stew

Ingredients

Serves 4

- 28 ounce can diced tomatoes (without onion or garlic)

- 20 greater massive shrimp (about 21-30/pound), peeled and deveined (tails may be left on); see word approximately cooking time if the use of frozen vs. Defrosted shrimp.

- 1 tablespoon dried basil

- 1 tablespoon garlic infused oil

- 2 cups baby kale leaves

- half of cup crumbled feta cheese

Instructions

1. In medium-big skillet, over medium heat, upload in diced tomatoes (consisting of any juice), shrimp, basil, garlic infused oil and simmer for two-three minutes or till shrimp are opaque and almost completely cooked.

2. NOTE: you can use frozen, peeled and deveined shrimp, however add every other 2-3 minutes to cooking time.)

3. When shrimp is pretty much fully cooked, add in infant kale leaves and feta, area cowl over skillet and allow mixture simmer for some other 2 mins or until kale continues to be brilliant inexperienced however wilted.

4. Serve in soup bowls.

5. Serving inspiration, serve stew as is or over a scoop of cooked rice or quinoa or perhaps with an appropriate crusty roll.

Roasted Greek Lemon Potatoes with Seared Chicken

Ingredients

Serves 4

- 3 massive Yukon gold potatoes (approximately 1 1/2-1 3/4 pounds)

- 1 half cups low FODMAP fowl broth (I used FODY food emblem)

- 1/3 cup freshly squeezed lemon juice (approximately 2 lemons)

- 1 teaspoon dried oregano

- 1/three cup + 1 tablespoon garlic infused oil

- 1 teaspoon salt

- pepper, to taste

- 1 pound hen cutlets(boneless/skinless), four pieces

- Optional garnish: lemon slices, sparkling oregano or parsley

Instructions

1. Preheat oven to 400 levels F.

2. Skin potatoes and cut into chunk size wedges

3. Add potatoes to rimmed baking sheet.

4. In bowl, add fowl broth, lemon juice, dried oregano, 1/3 cup garlic oil, salt and pepper, whisk to mixture.

5. Pour lemon combination over potatoes. Add a tented piece of aluminum foil over potatoes (prevents splattering) and vicinity in oven to roast for half-hour.

6. Meanwhile in skillet, upload last 1 tablespoon of garlic oil over medium warmness. Sear the chook on each facets to brown but do not prepare dinner

through, approximately 2-three mins in step with aspect.

7. Remove hen from skillet and set aside.

8. After the half-hour of roasting time for potatoes, use spatula to lightly flip the potatoes and cast off aluminum foil.

9. Add the hen to the rimmed baking sheet alongside the potatoes and prepare dinner for another 20 mins or till potatoes are fork tender and hen is cooked through (the use of a meat thermometer, cooked hen temperature is a hundred sixty five tiers F).

10. If preferred, garnish with sparkling parsley, clean oregano, and lemon slices.

Roasted Chickpea Tacos

Ingredients

Serves 6-eight, serving length 2 tacos

- 1, sixteen ounce can chickpeas, tired and rinsed

- half teaspoon Casa de Santé Chili Seasoning Mix

- 1 teaspoon garlic infused oil

- sea salt, to flavor

- 12-16 (soft) corn tortillas

Toppings:

- 2 cups baby lettuce veggies

- 1 pink pepper, deseeded and sliced into bite length pieces

- 1 inexperienced pepper, deseeded and sliced into chunk length pieces

- half cup lactose loose bitter cream (or sub in undeniable Greek yogurt, in case you tolerate it)

- half cup finely shredded Cheddar Jack cheese

- 1/4 cup cilantro, chopped, non-compulsory

- 1 fresh lime, sliced into wedges

Instructions

1. Preheat oven to 375 degrees F.

2. Add chickpeas to a rimmed baking sheet.

3. Using paper towel, dry off any liquid from chickpeas.

4. Add chili seasoning, oil and sea salt to chickpeas.

5. Using basting brush, unfold seasoning and olive over chickpeas.

6. Roast chickpeas in preheated oven on middle rack for 15 minutes, stirring after approximately 6 mins of cooking time.

7. Add tortillas to backside rack in oven to heat, about 2 mins on every side or heat up in a massive skillet over medium heat until each side of the tortilla is lightly browned but the tortilla continues to be pliable.

8. To serve, layer approximately 1/4 cup lettuce, followed via 1-2 tablespoons chopped pink and green pepper, a dollop of lactose free bitter cream, a sprinkle of cheese, 2 tablespoons roasted chickpeas, cilantro, if the usage of, followed by way of a squeeze of sparkling lime juice.

Roasted Tomatoes, Shrimp and Zoodles

Ingredients

Serves 4

- four cups spiralized zucchini (approximately three small zucchinis, ~100 gms every)

- 2/3 cup grape tomatoes

- three tablespoons pine nuts

- 2 tablespoon garlic infused oil

- 20 extra massive shrimp, peeled and deveined

- 1 tablespoon olive oil

- 1 tablespoon parmesan cheese (plus extra for garnish, if preferred)

- Pinch of red pepper flakes (about 1/4 teaspoon), non-obligatory

Instructions

1. Preheat oven to 375 stages F.

2. Layer zoodles, grape tomatoes,and pine nuts onto rimmed baking sheet.

3. Drizzle zoodles with garlic infused oil; using basting brush, brush oil evenly over zoodles.

4. Bake in oven for 20 mins, till tomatoes simply start to pop open and are fork gentle and zoodles are pliable.

5. While zoodles bake, stir fry shrimp in medium skillet over medium warmth with olive oil, for about 3 mins. When shrimp is opaque and cooked thru, sprinkle with Parmesan cheese and pink pepper flakes, if the usage of, and take away from heat.

6. When zoodles and tomatoes are performed, layer them into serving bowls or on a serving platter. Top with cooked shrimp and a sprinkle of Parmesan cheese, if preferred.

Seared Salmon Asian Inspired Nourish Bowl

Ingredients

Per Salmon Nourish Bowl

- 1 cup cooked pink rice (can sub in cooked quinoa, jasmine or basmati rice)

- four yellow bell pepper strips

- four red bell pepper strips

- 1 radish, sliced

- 1 cup finely chopped kale

- 1/2 cup sliced red cabbage

- 1/4 cup sliced carrots

- 1 tablespoon sliced inexperienced onion/scallion (green element most effective)

Optional garnish:

- 2 tablespoons chopped salted peanuts

- 1 tablespoon chopped mint and/or cilantro

- 4.Five ounce salmon filet

- Salt, pepper to flavor

- 1 teaspoon sesame oil

- 1/4 teaspoon sesame seeds, garnish (optional)

- Asian Dressing

- 2 teaspoon soy sauce

- 1 teaspoon rice wine vinegar

- 1 teaspoon chile paste (without garlic and onion- I used Union Foods Brand)

- 2 teaspoons sesame oil

- 1-2 teaspoons water

Instructions

1. In grill pan over medium warmth, upload sesame oil.

2. Prepare salmon with the aid of seasoning with salt, pepper and sesame seeds, if the use of.

3. Place salmon flesh aspect down in pan for 6 mins. Flip over and prepare dinner for some other 3 minute or till salmon is cooked thru and flakey, set aside. (Cooking time might also vary relying on thickness of salmon filet)

Assemble Nourish bowl:

1. Add warm rice to serving bowl and layer veggies around the rice in decorative sample (of path, which is as much as you!)

2. Add seared salmon to pinnacle of veggie/rice in bowl.

3. Drizzle with Asian dressing

4. Top with chopped nuts and herbs as
   preferred.

Santé Fe Tomato Lime Chicken (FODMAP
pleasant)

Ingredients

- 1 lb boneless skinless chook breast

- salt and pepper

- 1 garlic clove

- 2 TB oil

- 1, 14.5 oz. Can diced tomatoes (FODMAP
  followers test components)

- 1 small yellow pepper, deseeded and
  chopped

- 1 small bunch scallions, chopped (FODMAP fans use inexperienced part handiest) -about 1/3 cup

- 1 big lime juiced (use approximately 2 TB juice)

- 1/4 tsp Chipotle chili powder (FODMAP fans I do now not recognize if that is low- may additionally delete or check tolerance)

- half of cup shredded component skim mozzarella cheese

- 2 TB chopped clean cilantro or basil to garnish *optionally available

Instructions

1. In massive skillet warmness the olive oil over medium warmth and upload garlic clove to season oil.

2. Remove garlic.

3. Season bird with salt and pepper and cook about 3-4 mins every facet to brown the meat, but now not cook thru.

4. Add tomatoes, diced pepper and scallions to crock pot this is set on low placing.

5. Top with lime juice and chipotle seasoning if the use of and deliver a gentle stir.

6. Place browned chook on top of greens.

7. Cover slow cooker and cook for approximately 3 hours on low.

8. Take 2 forks and shred chook.

9. Sprinkle mozzarella cheese over the shredded fowl and replace cover on sluggish cooker for five mins--cheese must melt right up!

10. Garnish with sparkling herbs if desired.

Mediterranean Rice Salad

Ingredients

- Serves four (restriction to 1/4 cup chickpeas in step with serving for low FODMAP removal diet)

- 2/3 cup chopped flat leaf parsley

- 2 tablespoons chopped clean mint leaves

- 10 grape tomatoes, cut in quarters

- 2 tablespoons clean squeezed lemon juice

- 1 cup canned chickpeas, drained and rinsed

- 2 cups cooked brown rice (can sub in cooked quinoa)

- 1/4 cup olive oil

- Salt and pepper, to flavor

Instructions

1. Add substances to a medium size bowl, stir to blend.

2. Enjoy at room temperature or cool.

MEAL PLANS & SHOPPING LIST

Meal plan

Sunday

- Breakfast: Omelet with cheddar cheese, bell peppers, spinach, olives and tomatoes, gluten-loose toast with lactose free unfold, coffee.

- Lunch: Sandwich made with gluten-free bread, turkey (no HFCS), swiss cheese, alfalfa sprouts, HCFS-free mayonnaise and mustard. Corn chips, snack, sunflower, seedsGlass of lemonade.

- Dinner: Roast red meat, potatoes baked with salt and rosemary, salad made with lettuce and tomatoes and no HFCS balsalmic vinegar dressing, a tumbler of vulnerable peppermint tea.

Monday

- Breakfast: Smoothie made with banana, frozen strawberries, flax seeds and almond milk, inexperienced tea.

- Lunch: Sandwich made with gluten-loose bread, leftover roast beef, swiss cheese, mayonnaise and alfalfa sprouts, gluten-free crackers, snack, cantaloupe, glass of lemonade.

- Dinner: Baked fowl cooked with the spring-green a part of an onion, sunflower seed cooking oil, salt, pepper and topped with a HCFS sauce to serve, brown rice, steamed green beans with sliced almonds.

Tuesday

- Breakfast: Oatmeal with blueberries and brown sugar, espresso.

- Lunch: Leftover baked fowl, salad made with spinach, tomatoes, mandarin oranges and a raspberry (HCFS unfastened), French dressing, gluten free crackers, snack, sunflower seeds, glass of limeade.

- Dinner: Pork stir-fry made with cabbage, carrots, water chestnuts, bamboo shoots and inexperienced beans, brown rice, peppermint tea.

Wednesday

- Breakfast: Smoothie made with banana, frozen blueberries, chia seeds and almond milk, coffee.

- Lunch: Salad made with spinach, tomatoes, almond slices, tuna, and a raspberry (HCFS loose) French dressing, snack. Lactose-unfastened yogurt with strawberries, cup of vulnerable black tea.

- Dinner: Beef stew made with allowed ingredients, i.e. Parsnips (no tomato paste or onions).

Thursday

- Breakfast: Oatmeal with banana slices, almond milk and brown sugar, coffee.

- Lunch: Sandwich made with gluten-loose bread, turkey (no HFCS), swiss cheese, alfalfa sprouts, HFCS-free, mayonnaise and mustard, snack, cantaloupe, limeade.

- Dinner: Chicken adobo made with none of the meals to keep away from, gluten-free chips, salsa made with tomatoes, onion, veggies, parsley and limes, and cup of peppermint tea.

Friday

- Breakfast: Smoothie made with banana, frozen strawberries, flax seeds and almond milk, cup of espresso.

- Lunch: Gluten-free chips with melted cheddar cheese, diced tomatoes, bell peppers and olives, snack, leftover gluten-unfastened chips and salsa, limeade.

- Dinner: Pan-fried shrimp cooked in sunflower oil, topped with lemon, brown rice, stir fry vegetables: carrots, cabbage, green beans, and bean sprouts.

Saturday

- Breakfast: Gluten-loose waffles included with blueberries and maple syrup (made and not using a HFCS), cup of espresso.

- Lunch: Salad made with lettuce, bell pepper, tomato, alfalfa sprouts and topped with HFCS-unfastened dressing, snack, lactose-unfastened yogurt with strawberries, and cup of vulnerable black tea.

- Dinner: Baked ham slices crowned with pineapple chunks, potatoes baked in sunflower seed oil, salt, and rosemary leaves, baked green beans crowned with almond slices.

A Sample Low-FODMAP Shopping List

Many meals are clearly low in FODMAPs. Here is a simple shopping listing to get you began.

- Protein: Beef, chook, eggs, fish, lamb, pork, prawns and tofu

- Whole grains: Brown rice, buckwheat, maize, millet, oats and quinoa

- Fruit: Bananas, blueberries, kiwi, limes, mandarins, oranges, papaya, pineapple, rhubarb and strawberries

- Vegetables: Bean sprouts, bell peppers, carrots, Choy sum, eggplant, kale, tomatoes, spinach and zucchini

- Nuts: Almonds (no more than 10 consistent with sitting), macadamia nuts, peanuts, pecans, pine nuts and walnuts

- Seeds: Linseeds, pumpkin, sesame and sunflower

- Dairy: Cheddar cheese, lactose-unfastened milk and Parmesan cheese

- Oils: Coconut oil and olive oil

- Beverages: Black tea, espresso, inexperienced tea, peppermint tea, water and white tea

- Condiments: Basil, chili, ginger, mustard, pepper, salt, white rice vinegar and wasabi powder

- Additionally, it's critical to test the components listing on packaged foods for added FODMAPs.

- Food corporations may additionally upload FODMAPs to their foods for lots motives, consisting of as prebiotics, as a fats replacement or as a lower-calorie alternative for sugar.

- Many foods are evidently low in FODMAPs. That said, many processed meals have delivered FODMAPs and have to be restrained.

CONCLUSION

FODMAPs are short-chain carbs that move thru your intestines undigested. Many foods that include FODMAPs are considered very healthful, and a few FODMAPs feature like wholesome prebiotic fibers, helping your friendly intestine microorganism.

Therefore, folks who can tolerate these sorts of carbs need to no longer keep away from them. However, for humans with a FODMAP intolerance, ingredients high in those carbs may also motive ugly digestive problems and ought to be removed or constrained.

If you often enjoy digestive disillusioned that lowers your best of existence, FODMAPs ought to be in your list of pinnacle suspects. Though a low-FODMAP diet might not remove all digestive troubles, chances are high that it is able to cause considerable enhancements.

The low-FODMAP weight-reduction plan can dramatically enhance digestive signs, which include those in people with IBS. However, not everyone with IBS responds to the food regimen. What's greater, the weight-reduction plan entails a three-stage process which could take up to six months. And unless you want it, the weight loss program may also do more harm than correct, on

the grounds that FODMAPs are prebiotics that

help the boom of beneficial microorganism in

your gut.

This food plan may be used as a brief application

to discover meals that trigger pain. Once you've

finished the food plan, you will be capable of

pinpoint which high-FODMAP meals are tolerable

or triggering for you. This will let you make meals

alternatives that encourage you to sense you're

nice.

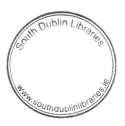

South Dublin Libraries
www.southdublinlibraries.ie

CPSIA information can be obtained
at www.ICGtesting.com
Printed in the USA
LVHW032337071220
673554LV00020B/4150